Sabbath Moments

Finding Rest for the Soul
in the Midst of Daily Living

Sabbath Moments

Finding Rest for the Soul in the Midst of Daily Living

Adolfo Quezada

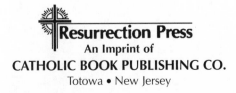

Resurrection Press
An Imprint of
CATHOLIC BOOK PUBLISHING CO.
Totowa • New Jersey

For

Maria, Cristina, Miguel

—··—··—··—··—··—··—··—

First published in February 2003 by Resurrection Press, Catholic Book Publishing Company.

Copyright © 2003 by Adolfo Quezada

ISBN 1-878718-80-0

Library of Congress Catalog Card Number: 2002115856

Cover design by Beth DeNapoli

Printed in Canada.

1 2 3 4 5 6 7 8 9

Acknowledgments

I am grateful to Emilie Cerar, the editor of Resurrection Press. She sees possibilities and pursues them. What is more, she has consistently challenged me to go beyond the norm and to reach for possibilities too. I am indebted to Emilie for believing in my work and for her editing skills that always make it better. I thank Melanie Supan Sethney for her timely insights and suggestions to the manuscript. I am especially grateful to me wife, Judy Quezada, whose constant support and encouragement have sustained me through the years and whose sharp eye and sensitive heart have helped guide my words.

"The Lord is my shepherd, I shall not want . . ."

> All that I need, I have been given, my sole
> desire is to be with God;

". . . he makes me lie down in green pastures . . ."

> God carries me away from the demands
> of a frantic world and lays me gently on the
> earth from which I come.

"He leads me beside still waters . . ."

> God calls me forth unto the deep
> restful waters of my spirit;

". . . he restores my soul . . ."

> God breathes new life into my being, and
> I am made whole again.

Contents

Foreword

A REFLECTIVE person welcomes any invitation away from chaos. *Sabbath Moments* is such an invitation. The title refers to a reality that can be both reachable and rare. In a fast paced consumer society where time spent without profit is seen as time wasted, the notion of time as gift, as rest, as opportunity to restore balance, becomes an inadmissible expense. The truth, however, is that what appears to be a luxury is really more necessary than other pursuits and possessions.

What is of greater value than self-knowledge, prayer and compassion? These are the fruits of a life grounded in God. They are fostered by attention to God's gifts surrounding us. One of those gifts is the biblical notion of Sabbath. On hearing that word we might readily think of a day kept holy by observant Jews. Wherever they live in large numbers their observance is visible. Shops close, special garb is worn and special food is served. They can be seen walking to temple and synagogue and visiting with one another. There is a saying that the Jews keep the Sabbath and the Sabbath keeps the Jews. The rabbis teach that Sabbath is a time of equality between rich and poor. The poor are free of labor on that day and share the same dignity as the rich. Sabbath is a time for evaluating one's work and for questioning its worth. Is what we do good for others, for the world, for ourselves? Further, Sabbath invites reflection on life itself. How competitive, how petty, how sensible, how realistic is my living? What is my relationship to others and to God?

As serious as it sounds, Sabbath is not solemn. The prophet Isaiah names it "a delight." He promises a rich reward for its observance. "If you refrain from trampling the Sabbath, from pursuing your own interests on my holy day; if you call the Sabbath a delight and the holy day of the Lord honorable; I will make you ride upon the earth; I will feed you with the heritage of your ancestor Jacob, for the mouth of the Lord has spoken" (Is 58, 13-14).

The point of this book is not about one day's observance but about the thread of Sabbath woven through one's week. The author's approach is realistic in that he lives the life of his readers and knows the many claims on their time. He is also practical in his counsel which is brief and down-to-earth. "What we are depends on what the Sabbath is to us," wrote Abraham Joshua

Heschel. One feels sure the Rabbi would celebrate Adolfo Quezada's insightful work for its profoundly simple grasp of the place of Sabbath in daily living.

Paul Curtin, C.Ss.R., Director
Desert House of Prayer
Tucson, Arizona

Preface

Sometimes, in the process of living, we forget to live. We are so busy *doing* that we forget *being.* The pace of our life keeps us from stopping long enough to let our soul catch up with us.

We are called to enter Sabbath Moments
where we can be still and know that God is God.

We try so hard to balance our responsibilities at home, at work, and in our social environment. We dedicate ourselves to taking care of others, and completing all our jobs. The demands placed on us by ourselves and others keep us moving like a roller coaster. And, rather than help us to slow down, technology provides a way to do things faster so we can accomplish even more.

We are called to enter Sabbath Moments
where we can rest and recreate.

At the end of the day we are exhausted and drained. We collapse in front of a television or computer screen to rest, but this is not restful; it only numbs our bruised and battered soul.

We are called to enter Sabbath Moments
where we can be restored.

In Hebrew, the word for "Sabbath" means a time of rest. It means freedom from activity or labor, from the busyness of life. Rabbi Abraham Heschel said that the idea of the Sabbath is to sanctify time, not so much to create space, but as a way to encounter the holy.

> *Let us enter into Sabbath Moments.*
> *Let our hearts abide in peace.*
> *Let us leave the crowd*
> *and cease our labor even for a while.*

First Week

Being God-Conscious

Day 1

✳ *Being Present* ✳

"When a man can suffer injustice
and endure hardship through his
awareness of God's presence, this
is the work of grace in him."
(1 Pet 2:19)

What does it mean to be "God-conscious"? It means that we are aware of the moment before us, and that we allow our senses to expose creation to us. It means that we experience God in all that is, including those with whom we interact. It means that we encounter God, even in the midst of our suffering. It means that we acknowledge the energy of God moving through us, defining who we are and animating what we do.

It seems so simple when we talk about living consciously; yet, many of us live out our lives as though we were asleep. Sometimes our mind is taken captive by obsessive thoughts. When this happens we are simply not available to life. We may go through the motions and we may act automatically; yet, we are in a trance-like state.

Our reactive emotions may also abduct us from the present. We are anxious about what might happen in the future; we feel guilty about what has happened in the past. And when it is too painful to stay in the past, the future, or the present, we enter the half-dead state of depression.

We are beings who think and feel; yet, even as we pay attention to our thoughts and respect our feelings, in God–consciousness we do not allow our thoughts or our feelings to take us away from the here and now.

I awaken to what is in the moment before me.
Here and now you are with me,
I dare to stay and relish your presence.
Let me abide with you forever.

Day 2

✳ *Embracing the Moment* ✳

"Now is the accepted time!
Now is the day of salvation!"
(2 Cor 6:12)

Life is the moment at hand, all else is memory or imagination. We can cherish our yesterday and anticipate tomorrow, but the moment before us is the crux of our reality. Sabbath Moments bring us into the reality of now. These are times of presence in which we are fully conscious of life; moments in which we love and are loved. It is in the present time of Sabbath Moments that we realize how the past has impacted on us and consider what the future might bring. When we pay attention to the moment at hand, we bring to it the benefit of our full consciousness. The gift of life is in the moment. God gives us all that we need to handle what is before us. We focus on what we can do now, what we can experience now, what we can realistically expect from ourselves now. Our responsibility is to take the present and to live it fully.

Living in the present moment, we face our poverty, and we are compelled to be honest about ourselves. When we leave the present we can easily forget our connectedness with God. In the present we make ourselves available to God. We learn to be dependent on God and to trust in that over which we have no control. Our soul lives in present time. The Eternal Now is all we have; it is where our soul meets God. We cannot cling to the moment before us, but we can fill it with love before we commend it to eternity.

My mind may fly to future times or
lag behind in memories, yet I can
only know you in the moment
that I find before me.

Day 3

✳ *Loving Consciously* ✳

"Remain here and stay awake with me."
(Mt 26:38)

To live consciously is to live deliberately, that is, with purpose and meaning. It is to drink in the wonder of creation through our senses and to unleash the divine creativity that finds its expression through us.

We were born into the world to give and receive love on behalf of God. We are here because it is "here" that we are at one with God. When we dare to remain here and stay awake with God, we are able to live our moment fully and with fecundity.

Conscious living means conscious loving. This begins with love for ourselves. As we love and honor our physical selves, we strive for the physical welfare of others. As we respond to our own emotional needs, we respond to the emotional needs of others. As we open ourselves to the realm of the spirit, we encourage others to be open as well.

When we remain here and stay awake with God we are able to use our gifts and talents effectively, including our ability to think and feel. Above all, when we remain here and stay awake with God, we allow God to live through us according to our uniqueness.

We are asked by God to stay this hour, this Sabbath Moment, in God-consciousness, awake to all that is, embracing the reality that is set before us.

You awaken me to the reality of now.
You bring me back from my evading slumber to
the consciousness of life. When my eyes grow
weary and I choose to escape, touch me with
your loving hand, that I may stay with you.

Day 4

✳ Resting the Soul ✳

"Come to me, all who labor and are
heavy laden, and I will give you rest . . ."
(Mt 11:28)

Tired and weary, overwhelmed and overburdened, we are bent over with the heaviness of life. We carry great responsibilities and are weighed down with the problems of the world. Then we are lured by the sweet and gentle voice of our Beloved to enter into rest.

The invitation to come and be restored is an invitation to enter Sabbath Moments throughout our day. It is not enough to rest our body; we must also rest our soul. We come to God and leave behind all that we have taken upon ourselves. We release our hold on the reins of control and shoulder the yoke of love. Here, we do not work alone but with God who shares the yoke. The yoke of love is easy and the burden of life is light. We listen to the rhythm of God's heart. The anxious, rapid beating of our heart gives way to God's slow and steady, strong and loving pulse.

*The yoke that binds us together
is a bond of souls. So are
we bound, that our life is one.
We are wedded into I Am.*

Day 5

✳ *Being Absorbed* ✳

*"Take my yoke upon you, and learn from me;
for I am gentle and humble in heart,…"*
(Mt 11:29a)

In Sabbath Moments we are taken beyond ourselves to something that intrigues us, absorbs us, and otherwise enraptures us. It may be the Divine Being whom we touch in prayer or it may be the antics of a hummingbird that fascinate us. Whatever the object of our attention, it is ecstatic in that it takes us out of ourselves, even momentarily.

Sabbath Moments are more than a time for doing; they are a time for being. In Sabbath Moments we are more open to our spirit and more accepting of our soul. This is not a time for thinking and sorting things out but for allowing God-consciousness; not so much for mental well-being, as for the well-being of our soul. Sabbath Moments are not a place to hide. We do not go there to escape life but to enter into it. It is here that we allow ourselves to be healed by the tender and accepting ways of God.

Sabbath Moments are our place of belonging, our refuge, our retreat. It is from here that we can launch ourselves into the world to do love's bidding. From Sabbath Moments we emerge refreshed and ready to live life fully, no matter what comes with it.

I am lifted away from that which
tethers me to chaos and confusion.
With single-heart I gaze upon the
beauty of what you lay before me.

✳ *Easing Our Work* ✳

"…and you will find rest for your souls."
(Mt 11:29b)

The rest that is promised is not without responsibility. As we take the yoke of love and wear it, we are joined to the power of God. We learn from God to move gently and with humility. We discover that it is not our brute force that propels our journey, but our union with that which is divine. We find rest for our soul, even in the midst of our labor. Yoked to the holy spirit of God, our soul bears the burden of life with ease.

Benedict of Nursia, the founder of Western mysticism, advocated a balanced life, and he included in his "Rule" the practice of prayer, study, work, and rest.

Rest is imperative in the work of creation and co-creation. Sabbath Moments are the spaces between bursts of energy, the silences between words spoken, the deaths between times of living. Without stopping to rest, to gather ourselves, and to remember who we are, we will live without purpose, direction, or meaning. We need some time to catch our breath. We need time to nourish our body with food and drink, and we need time to frolic and play. In Sabbath Moments we rest, restore, and recreate. Most important, when we enter Sabbath Moments, we break out of our routine and become conscious of God.

You call me into your midst to rest and
gather the myriad pieces of my life, to
regain the integrity which I have squandered
and to allow the consciousness of love.

Day 7

✳ *Learning from the Soul* ✳

". . . for my yoke is easy, and my burden is light."
(Mt 11:30)

Our soul is the seat of wisdom, a wisdom acquired from life itself—from entering into the experiences that occur along the journey. From our soul we learn about ourselves, about our needs and our internal resources. If we stay and listen to the wisdom of our soul, we are given all that we need to see us through the day. At one with our soul, we are understood and forgiven; we are welcomed home. At one with our soul, we are connected to all that is.

In Sabbath Moments our soul brings light into darkness, forcing us to slow down, pay attention, and live consciously. In the darkness, we have to fall back on intuition and instinct. We count on an inner knowing, rather than on concrete knowledge. In the darkness, it is not our intellect that helps us but our faith. Our soul takes us to our most inward place, our essence, our core. It is here, in the darkness, that we see the light.

28

You soothe and nourish me. You are the balm of my life, even in the worst of times. You touch me and ease the journey before me. You turn the hard, dry, and barren ground of my being into a yielding, moist, and fertile land.

Second Week

Allowing Rest

✳ Facing Ourselves ✳

*"So then, there remains a Sabbath
rest for the people of God; . . ."*
(Heb 4:9)

We will do almost anything it seems, to run away from
who we really are. We fear facing our basic self because we
believe in the illusion of separateness and finiteness. We
are afraid of our mortality and our aloneness. Unless we
have come to believe in the eternal oneness of all, we look
for diversion; we keep busy; we drug our mind; we work
nonstop—anything to avoid facing the starkness of our
reality. To escape the existential loneliness that we sometimes experience, we engage in frantic activity and pre-
tend to live a meaningful life. We pollute our senses, and
we seek fulfillment through addictive practices.

We are afraid to stop and be quiet because to do so we
would have to let go of the external dependencies which
we have come to know so well, and, instead, turn to the
internal dependencies which we know hardly at all. If we

were to stop, if we were to be quiet and contemplate the reality of our being, then we would have to acknowledge our nothingness, to feel our emptiness, and to enter into our darkness. This we dare not do lest we be reminded of our death. In our flight from our true selves, we run into the arms of a false and deceptive world—a world that promises to anesthetize us from the pain of living but which actually contributes to our anguish.

Liberate me from the distractions on which I am dependent. Grant me the courage to stop and rest, be still and pray, that I may face the Reality of my life.

Day 2

✳ *Stopping the Busyness* ✳

*" for whoever enters God's rest also ceases
from his labors as God did from his."
(Heb 4:10)*

Sometimes our sense of inadequacy keeps us working furiously lest others discover just how inadequate we feel we are. Sometimes we refuse to honor Sabbath Moments because we don't want to lose the momentum that we have built up doing whatever it is we are doing. We are afraid that if we stop, even for a moment, we may never get started again. Our habit to keep busy is hard to break, especially when our culture urges us to do more and more.

We may also be afraid that if we allow ourselves to enter into Sabbath Moments, we may have to confront our wounds and our grief which we have been holding at bay by means of our distractions and busyness. Sometimes we are afraid of what might come up from our deep unconscious if we create an opening. So, we press on with our busyness because it seems the safest place for us to be.

others all the time. Our service to others must be balanced with self-care.

*Even as I enter into the quiet hour
and ascend the mount to pray, I am
ready to descend into the valley
where needs compel my presence.*

Day 5

✳ *Offering Respite* ✳

*"…I assure you, as often as you did it for
one of my least brothers, you did it for me."*
(Mt 25:40)

We benefit from Sabbath Moments and want others to
benefit from them as well. As we offer respite and hospi-
tality to others in the name of God, we offer it to God.
Genesis tells the story of Abraham who was unknowingly
visited by God in the form of three strangers. Abraham
ran to greet them, saying, "Let some water be brought,
that you may bathe your feet, and then rest yourselves
under the tree…let me bring you a little food that you
may refresh yourselves, and afterward, you may go on
your way" (Gen 18:2-5). This is the way of love, to offer
Sabbath Moments to those who travel long, work hard,
and otherwise occupy themselves with the serious busi-
ness of living. And little do we realize that our restorative
gesture toward the least of our brethren is equally a gesture toward God.

Your will becomes my will. I am your sight, your voice, your touch. I am your presence and your love. Send me to the suffering; send me to the dying; send me to the poor and lost. Even as I rest and pray, I am ready to respond.

Day 6

❋ Revering the Sacred ❋

"One thing I ask of the Lord; this I seek: to dwell in the house of the Lord all the days of my life . . ."
(Ps 27:4a)

When we remain here and stay awake, we are enamored with life itself and with the world in which we live. We behold the wildflowers growing in the meadow; we smell the desert rain; we hear the love song of the hummingbird. In God-consciousness we touch the softness of a baby's cheek and taste the sweetness of a kiss.

In Sabbath Moments our soul enters her glory in the garden of God. Here, we revere the sacred that is all around us. Rocks, trees, and rivers, these are the colors of grounded ecstasy. We are in awe of all creation: ants, worms, leaves, dirt, mountains, valleys, and sky. Sometimes, when we least expect it, we are privy to a glimpse of heaven on earth.

*It would have been enough to
grant me life without the miracle of
sight. Yet, through your grace I can
behold the wonderment of all.*

Day 7

✳ *Being One with All* ✳

*"...that I may gaze on the
loveliness of the Lord . . ."*
(Ps 27:4b)

Even as the dawn is breaking all around us, we may experience Sabbath Moments of silent solitude. This prompting of the heart can spark a faith that carries us through yet another hour. As we allow creation to be what it is, we find ourselves entering into it. We move from a relationship of the observer and the observed, to the intimacy of one.

Conscious of the oneness that is, we behold our being in the stars; we delight in our fragrance in the roses; we touch our essence in the waves. It is our song that the sparrows offer, and our savor in the bees' sweet honey. This is the paradox of creation: we are distinct, yet we are in union with All; we are a part, yet we are the Whole.

I call your name and I respond. Your heart is mine and I feel your compassion. I too am blest to know your joy. Your handiwork is glorious; your creatures are but One.

Third Week

Respecting Cycles

Day 1

✳ **Honoring Our Limitations** ✳

"That is what the Lord prescribed. Tomorrow is a
day of complete rest, the Sabbath sacred to the Lord."
(Ex 16:23)

We are cyclic creatures much as the sun and moon, the oceans and the seasons. We ebb and flow; we rest and move; we have our ups and downs. Just like our circadian rhythms regulate our alternating periods of sleep and wakefulness, we are also cyclically regulated during our waking hours. It is believed that our rhythm is such that we need to rest in one way or another at least every two hours. A fifteen or twenty-minute break is best, but, depending on what we do with it, even taking a two or three-minute break helps. When we disregard this law of nature, the penalty may be high.

When we overextend ourselves for a prolonged time, we burnout, that is, we become physically, emotionally, and mentally exhausted. Unless we return frequently to our source of replenishment, we may fall victim to dis-

ease. When we ignore the signals that our mind and body send us and fail to take our Sabbath Moments, fatigue begins to set in and our brain chemistry reacts to the stress. Our body moves into a fight or flight mode, and we get a surge of energy that feels like a "second wind." In reality, we are experiencing our stress hormones kicking in and carrying us beyond where we should go. As our mind and body begin to breakdown, we may fall into depression.

Grant me the humility to admit my
limitations and to live accordingly.
Let me hear the pleas of my mind and body
to stop and honor the sacred time of rest.

❊ *Balancing Our System* ❊

"Observe the Sabbath day,
to keep it holy . . ."
(Deut 5:12)

Ultimately, our refusal to give ourselves Sabbath Moments may result in physical and emotional illness. Sabbath Moments allow our physical system to balance our basic bodily functions, including our stress hormones. During restorative breaks we relax and regulate our digestive system. Our system distributes nutrients throughout our body and regulates our cells to grow. The restive state has a calming and quieting effect on us.

When we heed the call from our mind and body for a restorative break, we can avoid bad stress and fatigue. Rest helps to balance the hemispheres of our brain and our nervous system. Even the molecules within our cells can be replenished when we take a restorative break. As it does when we're asleep, our mind is allowed to reorganize and to make sense of our experiences and the emotions that result from them. From Sabbath Moments come new meaning and understanding about our life.

It is not enough that I act and move and have my being in you. You would also have me come to rest in the cradle of your love where I am restored, refreshed, and recreated.

Day 3

❈ *Receiving Restoration* ❈

"Therefore, you must keep the
Sabbath as something sacred."
(Ex 31:14)

We can learn about the ebb and flow of rest and action from our sister hummingbird. The vitality with which she moves comes from the enthusiasm of a soul in love with life. But always she knows to stop and rest, to stop and revitalize, to stop and be centered before she moves again. The hummer commits herself to be still longer than to be doing. She remembers her need to receive. She spends much time alone. At times she enters into torpor, there to be protected through the night and be restored for yet another day.

With the humility of the hummingbird, let us remember that we can move only because first we have stopped before God; we can work only because first we have rested with God; we can give only because first we have received from God; and we can love only because first we have been loved by God.

Rhythm of Life, I surrender to your pendulous ebb and flow. You thrust me forth to live with passion, then, hold me in abeyance to rest my weary soul, only to be cast out once again to live wholeheartedly.

Day 4

✳ *Listening to Our Bodies* ✳

"…I have stilled and quieted my soul
like a weaned child. Like a weaned child
on its mother's lap, so is my soul within me."
(Ps 131:2)

If we listen to ourselves, we will know when it is time for Sabbath Moments. We need to monitor ourselves because we are the only ones who know when it is time to stop. When we listen to the cues and dare to stop awhile, we discover that it is not just physical restoration that we need, but also spiritual reconnection. It is when we have become still and quiet that we hear God speak to us. It is the voice of a mother comforting her child, a father encouraging his child. In Sabbath Moments we hear the voice of God because we listen with our heart.

Our body will tell us when we are tired and in need of rest or sleep. If we become irritable and difficult to live with, our emotions are telling us to retreat and tend to ourselves with fun and relaxation. We may feel hungry for nourishment, or we may feel lonely and in need of the company of a friend. We may ignore our need for Sabbath Moments, but our mind, body, and soul do not.

As I respond to the needs of a child, let me also respond to my own. Help me to be sensitive to my need for rest and recreation, pause and restoration.

Day 5

✳ *Responding to Our Needs* ✳

*"For I will refresh the weary soul; every
soul that languishes I will replenish."*
(Jer 31:25)

How we spend our Sabbath Moments depends on what we know about ourselves in terms of what nourishes us, what is fun and relaxing to us, and what restores us. Each of us is different and needs different things at different times, but we have to slow down to recognize what it is we need. We may be in need of physical rest more than anything else. Perhaps we need to read or write. We may need community or we may need aloneness. While needs may vary from one person to another, one need that is common to all of us is the need to pray and communicate with God heart to heart. We may want to visit a quiet church on a weekday where we find sanctuary.

Sabbath Moments may include any activity or inactivity that replenishes our soul. We may take a bike ride or a walk in the park. We may dance to music or just sit and listen to it. We may watch a movie. We may want to play. The soul loves to play. Through play we are re-created. We are not children, yet, we can approach life in a childlike manner, daring to be spontaneous, not allowing public opinion to squash our fun-loving selves. "Trust me when I tell you that whoever does not accept the kingdom of God as a child will not enter into it" (Lk 18:17). In our playfulness, we are receptive to the unexpected and unplanned, and we are open to what comes.

Fill my heart with the spirit of childhood, and let my laughter imbue my world. Lift me from the mire of my seriousness, and grace me with the courage to frolic foolishly.

Day 6

✳ *Finding Breaks* ✳

"...there the weary are at rest."
(Job 3:17)

Regardless of our responsibilities, we can always find a block of time to call our own. It may be a half-hour lunch period, a fifteen-minute coffee break, or even a five-minute bathroom break, but it is up to us to take the time we are entitled to. We are our own worst taskmasters when we work through lunch or fail to take our breaks and to use them wisely. Some of us cram several errands into a lunch hour and eat on the run. A coffee break can be used socializing in the lounge or it can be used to take a solitary walk. A long vacation or retreat can be of great benefit to us, but sometimes the rest we need may come in small, frequent opportunities. Just a few Sabbath Moments can make a world of difference.

Sometimes the time for resting comes to us from out of nowhere. We miss a bus, we get stuck in traffic or must wait for a bank teller or grocery clerk to be free. These and

Fourth Week

Daring to Stop

Day 1

✳ Doing Nothing ✳

"Better is one handful with tranquility than
two with toil and a chase after the wind!"
(Eccl 4:6)

Parkinson's Law stipulates that "work expands so as to fill the time available for its completion." The demands of life do not respect our need to recreate. It seems demands grow in proportion to our willingness to meet them, regardless of our ability to do so. Letting go of the world and all it asks of us brings rest to our soul. Not one of us is so important, so indispensable, that we have no time for resting.

Thomas Merton once remarked that the hardest thing for us to do is to do nothing. Yet, nothing is exactly what we sometimes need to do. It takes a brave heart to set aside the grandiose expectations that we sometimes have for ourselves, and to just sit on a log and do absolutely nothing. It is at a time like this that the Eternal Now rises up to meet us. It is in these Sabbath Moments that God can approach us.

other such opportunities are bonus Sabbath Moments if we choose to respond to them in that way. Instead of seething because someone is late or has cancelled an appointment with us, we can use our time praying, journaling, or just watching people go by. Instead of becoming frustrated because the line we are waiting on is moving at a snail's pace, we can use our time in conscious breathing. These times may be seen as inconveniences or they may be received as gracious gifts.

Let me enter conscious living.
Awaken me to the time of action and
the time of rest. Prepare me for doing
as well as being, for work and for repose.

✳ **Planning Rest** ✳

"For six years you may sow your field, and for six years prune your vineyard, gathering in their produce. But during the seventh year the land shall have a complete rest, a Sabbath for the Lord, when you may neither sow your field nor prune your vineyard."

(Lev 25:3)

Sabbath Moments may not always come spontaneously. It may be necessary to schedule them into our day just like we do other appointments. They need to be a regular part of our daily living. Morning prayer, for example, done at the same time, in the same place, serves us well throughout the day. What is crucial here is that we prioritize our prayer and meditation time over everything else.

We do not have to wait until we are utterly drained and exhausted before we rest. Sabbath Moments taken before we are tired give us the alertness we vitally need to do our work. We can prevent fatigue by resting, rather than resting to alleviate fatigue. We do not rest so that we may be ready to go back to work. We rest because it is in our nature to stop our activity and restore our energies. Our psychic energy undergoes a constant death and resurrection. It breaks down and must be built up again.

We are not unlike the farmer's field that must lie fallow periodically in order to restore the lost elements and energy before it can be used again. Activity and dormancy depend on one another. Life is pulsation.

Grace of Heaven, Giver of Life,
you hold nothing back from me.
What I receive, I pass on to the
World; then, I return to you for more.

get complete rest from the activity that we do day in and day out.

You slow me down and sometimes bring me to a stop. You would have me catch my breath and watch the hummingbird. You want my attention.

Day 3

❈ Nesting for Creativity ❈

"But Martha was distracted with much serving; and she went to him and said, 'Lord, do you not care that my sister has left me to serve alone? Tell her then to help me.'"
(Lk 10:40)

In Sabbath moments we don't have to get anything done. We merely have to stop and behold what God has wrought. From our place of nesting, we may respond creatively. There are some things that we can only do if we are rested. Anything that requires creativity, for example, requires a rested body, mind, and spirit. In fact, creativity does not venture into chaotic, busy places, but instead is born in a calm and restful nest.

Of course we need to make a living and to do what we must do. We are responsible beings and our services are important. Yet, we are concerned about too many things, and only one is necessary. The work of Martha is vital and can never be ignored, but neither can we forget to do as Mary and stop to rest awhile.

hard for us to gather our thoughts, but we can gather pebbles from the ground. And when it seems that God is nowhere to be found, we settle for a hummingbird atop a desert tree.

When my heart is heavy and
I cannot stop to pray, let the
simple, plain, and ordinary be
my refuge and my base.

✳ Treading Turbulent Waters ✳

"…Hold Infinity in the palm of your
hand and Eternity in an hour."
—William Blake

Only days had passed since the death of my son and I tried in vain to pray. It was as if the well was dry and God was far away. I went to the backyard and watered the grass. "Don't let the grass die," I kept repeating as if it was a mantra. The cascading water from the hose, the thirsty lawn, these became my focus. I could not pray, but in that moment I could connect with the water and the grass. Somehow, that was enough for then.

Sometimes the prayer that comes is in the form of tears. Sometimes a sigh is all we have to give. In any case, what matters is not the manner of our expression but the expression in and of itself. At times when we are afraid or anxious of the unknown, we do not judge our feelings, but simply remind ourselves, "Whatever will be, I will handle it."

A sigh, a groan, a tear, a glance—
sometimes this is all I have to offer.
Accept the expression of my poverty;
receive the gifts of my empty prayer.

Day 7

✳ *Focusing on the Simple* ✳

*"Jesus bent down and started tracing
on the ground with his finger."*
(Jn 8:6)

In troubled times the nature of Sabbath Moments is raw and spontaneous. We stop and doodle on the margin of a book; we play with a loose string on our shirt; we clip our nails or polish shoes. Washing pots and pans is a great way to ground ourselves, whether or not we are doing it prayerfully. What matters is the focus on the small, the simple, and routine.

The psychic benefit of Sabbath Moments is not in their loftiness but in their ability to ground us in the reality before us and to take us away from that which overwhelms us. When the forest is more than we can handle, we focus on the trees. When even an hour seems like more than we can bear, we stay with Sabbath Moments.

Let me be about the one thing
necessary. Having stopped to
be with all that gives me life,
I can do what you require of me.

✳ Choosing the Good Portion ✳

*"But the Lord answered her, 'Martha, Martha,
you are anxious and troubled about many things;
one thing is needful. Mary has chosen the good
portion, which shall not be taken away from her.'"*
(Lk 10:41)

It is not a matter of choosing between action and contemplation. From contemplation we act in the name of
God, and from action we return to contemplation. This is
the *yin* and *yang* of life, the ebb and flow of our vital
forces. To serve the children of God is to serve God. But
to sit at the feet of our Beloved and listen to the truths that
fill our soul is essential for any action we may take. We will
not be anxious or troubled when our doing follows our
being. Let us choose the one thing that is needful—the
willingness to stop and rest our soul awhile as we listen to
God within.

We know, for example, that the Buddha was enlight-
ened after meditating under a tree for a long time, and
that Mohammed withdrew into a cave every year to seek

direction from within. Before beginning to teach and preach, Catherine of Siena spent three years in seclusion in which she had mystical experiences. Jesus, too, needed to go into the wilderness for many days and nights in order to receive the insights that were to launch his ministry. Whoever we are and whatever we do, we too must learn the lesson that something comes of nothing. When we allow the space and reserve the time for quiet germination, the nothingness of night gives birth to God's creation.

I dare to be idle, I dare to be still.
Lead me to the realm of nothingness
where all I have to do is be. All comes
from nothing and nothing becomes All.

✻ *Grounding Ourselves* ✻

*"To see a World in a Grain of Sand
and a Heaven in a Wild Flower, . . ."*
                                        —*William Blake*

There are times in our life when we can barely hold ourselves together. These may be times when we are facing great stressors, or when we are still reeling in the wake of a tremendous loss. Whatever the burden in our heart may be, we are so overwhelmed by it that we are in no mood to pray or to go within. Ironically, in these times when we most need to enter Sabbath Moments, that is the last thing on our mind. We are too busy just trying to make it through from one hour to the next.

In the midst of our chaos or confusion, sorrow or anxiety, we need to ground ourselves in concrete ways. This may not be a time for our usual prayer, but instead a time to notice the intricacies of a flower growing wild in a field. It may not be a time for our usual meditation, but instead a time to watch a colony of ants go by. Perhaps it is too

Fifth Week

Sabbath Solitude

Day 1

✳ *Being Alone* ✳

"Come with me by yourselves to
a quiet place and rest a while."
(Mk 6:31)

Leaving the place in which we normally spend our time and energy, and entering into a different environment helps us to open the window of self-understanding. In a place apart we touch the depths of our being to which we are oblivious in our busy life. In our solitude we are alone and unavailable to others. Solitude is a state of being alone with ourselves and with God. It is where we go to meet ourselves and discover who we are.

In Sabbath solitude we find our basic self. We face off with who we are and no one else. Left alone, we are compelled to be honest about everything. We know the truth about ourselves, and we cannot deny it anymore. In solitude we fall back on ourselves for support, care, encouragement, comfort, and companionship. There is no one to whom to look except ourselves. We are the one who must discern what to do in each and every case. In solitude, we are responsible for ourselves and for the way we live the moments of our life.

You ask me to leave the crowd
and venture to a place apart,
a place of quiet and placidity.
There I will be alone with you.

Day 2

✳ Retreating into Solitude ✳

"When he had sent them away, he went up on the mountain by himself to pray, remaining there alone as evening drew on."   *(Mt 14:23)*

In solitude we see ourselves through the eyes of God. We respond to the prompting of our truest self, not the whims and expectations of the world at large. In solitude we set aside the image of our life. There is no one to impress, no one we have to please. We discover what we feel and what we think, separate and apart from others. In raw and naked self-disclosure, we see ourselves for who we are.

Sixteenth Century essayist, Michel Montaigne, said, "We must reserve a little back-shop, all our own, entirely free, wherein to establish our own true liberty and principal retreat and solitude." The "back-shop" may be an actual physical location to which we can at times retreat in solitude. It also may mean the place in ourselves where we go mentally to be at peace and rest intellectually and emotionally.

To flee from intimacy or responsibility is not a good reason to seek solitude. The solitary state is a way of being, not a haven that protects us from the world. From solitude we are cast out among the people to share with them in public what we have received in private. Rather than seclude us from the troubles of the world, solitude will fortify us to re-enter the world with more zeal. Eventually, we must leave our solitude and re-enter the city once again, but now we bring new vision and an image of the Whole.

Blessed is the state of my aloneness, for it is here that the divine breaks through to the essence of my being. O Sabbath Solitude, you nurture me and give me strength. You strip me down and make me real.

Day 3

✳ Silencing the Mind ✳

"For God alone my soul waits in silence . . ."
(Ps 62:1)

In Sabbath Moments we invite the veil of silence to descend upon our heart. From the silence within the silence, we listen with our heart. It is here in this silent space which opens deep within that God abides waiting to be heard.

When we allow the quiet into our Sabbath Moments, the quiet permeates the other moments of our life. We find that we are more conscious of our deeper reality, even as the ordinary events of life preoccupy us.

Our tendency is to live in duality, that is, to allow our mind to be divided. This keeps us confused and scattered. Our mind is noisy when our attention is given away to multiple distractions. We silence our mind when we allow all of our attention to focus on the one thing necessary—the presence of God in our life. In Sabbath Moments we find a place in which we are free from distractions and

where silence is the order of the day. This is a place where time is for wasting and solitude is for relishing.

You sing to me in silence and you touch my deepest self. I listen for the space between the notes. Your quiescence resounds in my soul.

Day 4

✳ *Ceasing the Noise* ✳

*"It is good to hope in silence
for the saving help of the Lord"
(Lam 3:26)*

Silence is more than the cessation of words and noises. It brings peace to the thoughts, the desires, and the obsessions that plague our psyche. It dismisses the demands and expectations that chase our being. Our plans, our worries, and our memories are set aside. We quiet the noises of our inordinate ambition and quiet our need to know. We turn off the critical tapes of our past and the immobilizing anxieties about our future. The control we exert over our life is relinquished.

The silence that comes in Sabbath Moments cannot be induced by us alone. We cannot produce it at will, nor can we manage its depth. Silence does not come from our control of the external but from the humble abandonment of our inner self. It is by allowing God to take us into the silence that we can enter there.

Silent One, who lives within me, gracious are your ways. You offer me the gift of peace and the stillness of the night. In the quiet and tranquility my soul begins to hear.

Day 5

✳ Meditating on ✳ One Thing Only

"Blessed are the single-hearted,
for they shall see God."
(Mt 5:8)

In Sabbath Moments we can allow ourselves to enter into a meditative state. This means that we allow our mind to be focused on one thing and block out everything else. We allow this instead of forcing it because such effort only distracts us from our purpose. Ultimately, meditation is learning to do one thing at a time.

A simple step toward a meditative state is that of noticing our breath. For some, it helps to count the exhalations by fours. For others, it helps merely to be conscious of the breath and to gently return to that consciousness every time the mind is distracted by anything else.

Another way to enter into a meditative state is by becoming acutely aware of our body and our bodily movements. As we heighten the awareness of our breathing, our walking, our dancing, or of our physical meditative practices, such as Tai Chi, our bodily consciousness is awakened to the exclusion of anything else. Again, we end up doing just one thing at a time.

We can also enter a meditative state by focusing our sight and attention on a specific external object. Our focus is not passive but active. The result of concentrating on one object is that all else is shut out. In that meditative moment of focused attention, we are single-hearted.

To seek you with my whole being is the instinct of my soul. For this I was born: to remain with you in love and devotion through the darkness and the unknowing.

Day 6

✳ *Relaxing Deeply* ✳

"...Our Father in heaven,
hallowed be your name, . . ."
(Mt 6:9)

When we allow ourselves to enter into a meditative state it produces for us a physiological state of deep relaxation. Meditation results in a lower metabolic rate and decreases our heart and respiration rates. Even the pattern of our brain waves change in the meditative state. Though relaxed, in meditation we are awake and alert to life. It is as if we can delve more deeply into reality.

A mantra of one word or phrase may also serve as a reminder to return to our center. Repeating a mantra that holds a special meaning or significance, such as the name we call God, helps us to remember God, even in our busyness. We can also pray the Lord's Prayer or other short prayers in a rhythmical way, coordinating the words with our breath.

God of love, live through me.
God of life, love through me.
God of love, live through me.
God of life, love through me.

Day 7

✳ *Praying Always* ✳

"At every opportunity pray in the Spirit,
using prayers and petitions of every sort."
(Eph 6:18)

In Sabbath Moments we may remember God through external prayer. Some people use the "Jesus Prayer" to stay God-conscious during their daily activities. This consists of repeating the prayer over and over silently, even as one moves and acts in the world. The long version is, "Lord Jesus Christ, Son of the Living God, have mercy on me, a sinner." This can be shortened to "Lord Jesus, Son of God, have mercy on me," or just simply, "Jesus." Other short prayers can also be used in this way to gather ourselves.

Sometimes we need to actually talk with God in prayer. We can confess our errors, reveal our secrets, and give voice to our fears. We can sort out our thoughts and acknowledge our feelings in prayer. We can make our wishes known and, at the same time, declare our alle-

giance to the ultimate will of God. As we pray, we allow a harmonious state of mind and an integration of the warring elements within.

We may also choose to enter into contemplation through centering prayer. In conjunction with conscious breathing, we do progressive relaxation of our muscle groups, focusing on the various parts of the body, one at a time. Then we use the familiar, intimate name that we call God as a mantra, and this returns us to our breathing and to God-consciousness.

With single heart I journey home to you.
Time and again I become distracted and
confused; yet, time and again, you call
me back to my center where you abide.

Sixth Week

The Breath of God

❉ *Inhaling God* ❉

*"…the Lord God formed man out of the clay
of the ground and blew into his nostrils the
breath of life, and so man became a living being."*
(Gen 2:7)

Breath is life and life is God. As we receive the breath of God, we receive the spirit that animates our soul. But even as we inhale the Life Principle, which is the breath of God, we are apt to take our breath for granted, as well as our life. Since breathing comes automatically, we tend to be oblivious to it until something happens to block its natural flow. As necessary as breath is for the maintenance of life, we pay little or no attention to it. As we ignore our breath, we ignore God, who is its source. Let us awaken from our stupefied sleep and stay awake that we may respond to God's animation of our soul.

When we breathe unconsciously, we also live unconsciously. This means that we move through life disconnected from God and unaware of God's presence in every moment of our day. We can be relatively functional as we

perform our duties and routines, but this automatic living is not the conscious living to which we are called. As often as possible, let us pause and be mindful that we are breathing, and let us be conscious of God who is present in our every breath. Let us focus on our breathing even in the midst of our busy day.

Your breath ignites the life within me, and sustains me through my days. I breathe your breath and am united to the essence of all Life.

Day 2

❋ *Breathing Consciously* ❋

*"…the spirit of God has made me, the
breath of the Almighty keeps me alive"
(Job 33:4)*

Our breath links our body, mind, and spirit, and con-
nects our conscious self with our unconscious self.
Conscious breathing awakens us to our body. As we pay
attention to our breath, we notice our stomach rising and
falling, expanding and contracting. This is the same ebb
and flow that is present in all forms of life. It is the same
rhythmic pattern of the ocean tides and the alternating
cycles of day and night. Conscious breathing awakens us
to our mind. Our mind becomes sharper and more alert,
and it opens to possibilities yet unknown. Conscious
breathing awakens us to our spirit. Our breath takes us to
higher realms where we encounter the essence of ourselves. Here, we are quickened by the breath (spirit) of
God, and are sent out to live for God, with God, and in
God.

Even in this moment we can become aware of our breathing. We breathe in and we breathe out. We breathe in and we breathe out. Our breath keeps us alive, but awareness of our breath keeps us life-conscious. This means that we are present to this moment in our life, this reality, this opportunity. Breathing in makes us aware of our *yin* (feminine) energy through which we are open and willing to receive. Breathing out, we are aware of our *yang* (masculine) energy through which we pass on to the world that which we have been given. Together, our inhalation and our exhalation form the primordial breath, which is of God. We breathe in and we breathe out. With each inhalation we accept the gift of life. With each exhalation we put ourselves out into the world.

Breath of life, Spirit of God, you
quicken my soul. Our encounter
is the genesis of my becoming. The breath
we breathe, we breathe together.

Day 3

✳ *Invoking the Divine* ✳

"I myself…will go along to give you rest."
(Ex 33:14)

In Sabbath moments it is not enough to still our mind or to pray with words or gestures. We must also invoke the presence of the divine into our moments. Sabbath Moments return us to our essence where we are one with God.

In Sabbath Moments we take the journey home. Leaving the world behind, we enter into soul prayer, contemplating God and God alone. In soul prayer we stop speaking to God and just listen. We stop trying to connect with God and just allow union with the divine.

When lovers reunite after a long absence, they cling to each other and just hold on. Words are not necessary, in fact, at a time like this, they just get in the way. Such is our time of prayer and contemplation with God. Being away from God, even for a little while, seems too long. In God we rest and have our being.

*My soul yearns for
your simple presence.
My spirit dissolves in
your potent love.*

Day 4

✳ Communing with the Beloved ✳

"But for me, to be near God is my good . . ."
(Ps 73:28)

In soul prayer we let go of expectations and allow for what God wills. We desire neither special feelings nor the dawning of new light, we come simply to be with God. Our soul prays, our heart sings, we are in love with God. Here, in the presence of God, we know that we are loved beyond human measure. Here, in contemplation of God, we dare to stay, if only for a Sabbath Moment.

To be conscious of the immanence of God is to live in full abundance. This is our treasure of the heart: to be in communion with our Beloved, to know that we are one. All else is built on this foundation; that all is one, and one is all. But how easily we allow the illusion of our separate self, how quickly we forget the unity of our being.

And so we pray, for prayer is remembering. We remember that we are the life of God in the world. We remember that love is our language and compassion is our fruit. We remember that ephemeral is our name and eternal is our soul.

Can we be closer than our oneness?
Is there more intimacy than the unity
we share? Is there more wholeness
than our sacred indivisibility?

Day 5

✳ Commending Ourselves ✳ to God

"Enough, then, of worrying about tomorrow. Let tomorrow take care of itself."
(Mt 6:34)

But how are we to pray when our heart is full of worry, anger, and deceit? How do we remember when our mind is filled with noise?

In prayer we *surrender* and let go of our resistance to what is. No more do we try to control. We lay aside our armor and retreat from our defense. Our mind, our heart, our soul, and our strength are captured by Love's force. Into the hands of God we commend our vanquished self. We let our will be one with God's, and our purpose becomes clear: to be the light of the Divine for all the world to see.

In prayer we *awaken* to the moment that is now. We leave yesterday to memory and tomorrow to our dreams.

The eternal moment set before us is all we really have, yet, in this sacred moment is the power of all time. Consciously, we live our life; consciously, we love. To stay awake for just this moment is all we need to do. To stay awake in prayer is our vigil through the night.

I surrender into the fullness
of your moment. I hold nothing
back from you. My anxiety gives
way to the naughting of my soul.

Day 6

✳ *Depending on God* ✳

*"Only in God be at rest, my soul,
for from him comes my hope."*
(Ps 62:6)

In prayer we are *vulnerable,* we stand naked and alone. We dare to feel emotion and expose our truest self. With purity of spirit and the weakness of a lamb, we become dependent, totally in need. We are as a babe suckled at the breast of God. We are the desert waiting for the rain. All our thoughts of self-sufficiency have been laid to rest, and we no longer look to power for protection of our soul.

In prayer we are *emptied* of all that does not count. Only Spirit can fulfill us; only Love can fill our void. Filled to the brim with the superfluous, we feel an emptiness inside. Emptied of all that would enslave us, we are fulfilled indeed. In the paradox of prayer, letting go is to receive. The full shall be emptied, and the empty shall be filled.

I am but a babe surrendered in its mother's arms. You suckle me to give me life; you are my sustenance, my strength, my everything.

Day 7

✳ **Dying to Our False Selves** ✳

". . . unless the grain of wheat falls to the
earth and dies, it remains just a grain of
wheat. But if it dies, it produces much fruit."
(Jn 12:24)

In prayer we *die* to self that God may live. The mask of our pretension falls off the face of God. In this death and resurrection that occurs in deeper prayer, we are left in total darkness as we wait unto the light. There is nothingness around us; there is silence in our midst. We have died to an illusion; we are born into New Life.

In Sabbath Moments we are held in the divine womb of God wherein we are nurtured, restored, and prepared to enter into the world again. Then we break out of the shell of our fabricated self and let the essence of ourselves be born.

I come to you for solace and comfort, yet, you give me so much more. You give me the merging of rivers, the union of lovers, the yoking of spirits, and the oneness of One.

You Ask of Me a Moment

God of eternity, maker of time,
you ask of me a moment, a pause, a glance.

Yet, I dare not stop to be with you when
I am needed at the front. I must respond
to a frantic world; I have so much to do.

God of silence, bringer of peace,
you ask of me a moment, a stillness, a calm.

But my mind is racing and my heart beats fast,
as I tend to the noises that demand my all.

God of the Sabbath, fount of repose,
you ask of me a moment, a respite, a sigh.

Time is of the essence; the day is always
filled. Perhaps when all the work is done
I may take time to rest, perchance to pray.

God of love, tender of souls,
you wait for me until I come.

May I pause for you,
take a moment for you.
That's all you ask of me.

Other Books by the Author

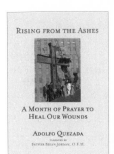

RISING FROM THE ASHES
A Month of Prayer to Heal Our Wounds
Adolfo Quezada

". . . helps the reader to heal spiritually and to ask God to give us hope in our present crisis."

—*Fr. Brian Jordan, OFM*

No. RP 158/04   Price: $4.95   CAN $7.95
ISBN 1-878718-72-X Size: 5" x 7"   48 pages

HEART PEACE
Embracing Life's Adversities
Adolfo Quezada

"This is one of the most authentic books I have ever read on the gut wrenching conditions that cause or lead to human suffering. . . . His book is a gift, allowing others to be the beneficiaries of his spiritual journey."   **—*Antoinette Bosco***

No. RP 117/04 Price: $9.95   CAN $15.95
ISBN 1-878718-52-5 160 pages Size: 5$\frac{1}{4}$" x 8$\frac{1}{4}$"

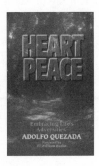

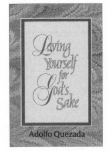

LOVING YOURSELF FOR GOD'S SAKE
Adolfo Quezada

This exquisite book of meditations gently directs the reader to see the gift of self in an entirely new and beautiful light. It presents a spirituality of self-love not based on narcissism, but as a response to the divine invitation to self-nurturing.

No. RP 720/04 Price: $5.95   CAN $9.55
ISBN 1-878718-35-5 96 pages Size: 4" x 6"

Additional Titles Published by Resurrection Press, a Catholic Book Publishing Imprint

For a free catalog call 1-800-892-6657
Visit our website: www.catholicbookpublishing.com

Day 4

✳ *Tending to Others* ✳

"...the Sabbath was made for man,
not man for the Sabbath. . . ."
(Mk 2:27)

Sometimes we must choose to go away to tend to our own needs before we can return to minister to others. Other times, however, we must choose to cut short our time of rest in order to respond to the needs of others.

In our scrupulosity we may sometimes lose the spirit of the Sabbath. To abstain from work and cease preoccupation in honor of the Sabbath does not abrogate our responsibility to others. We do our best to take time out and rest our soul; yet, we must be ready to respond to what life presents us. Even in the midst of Sabbath Moments we may be called upon to heal a brother, feed a sister, or clothe a child. In lovingkindness the letter of the law gives way to the spirit of the law. At the same time, humility keeps us mindful of our limitations. We cannot be everything to everybody, nor can we be available to apart from the crowd, even from our family and friends, to rest awhile.

Sabbath Moments, sacred time, I enter you with trepidation. Help me to know that I can come without great plans or expectations. Dare I leave my work behind to take a breath and rest awhile? Dare I open to the still point from whence comes my restoration?

Day 3

✳ *Absenting Ourselves* ✳

"Let us therefore strive to enter that rest . . ."
(Heb 4:11)

Some of us are caught up in the service of others and feel guilty leaving our ministry or family responsibility even for a little while because we believe we are needed constantly. Henri Nouwen wrote about the "ministry of absence." He believed that when we absent ourselves from those whom we serve, we give ourselves the opportunity to experience a special presence of God. Nouwen believed that our ministry of presence needs to be balanced by the ministry of absence. He believed that our primary vocation is not to be present to others in all their needs, but rather, it is, as it was for Jesus, to live constantly in the presence of God. From there we find the necessary balance from which to minister to others.

Sometimes we need to leave the place in which we live or work in order to enter Sabbath space. We have to go

Your nature is like the ocean. You ebb and flow; you wax and wane; you work and rest. Who am I to disallow the respite that my soul requires?

✳ *Interrupting Routine* ✳

*"...a woman named Martha received him (Jesus) into
her house. And she had a sister called Mary, who
sat at the Lord's feet and listened to his teaching."*
(Lk 10:38-39)

To dare to incorporate Sabbath Moments into our life,
we must also dare to go against the predominant opinion
that idleness is bad. We must be willing to interrupt the
momentum that builds up in our daily living, especially at
work, and stop to do little or nothing. We must be willing
to work hard and then, occasionally, not work at all; to
strive for excellence and then, occasionally, not strive at
all; to be productive and then, occasionally, not to produce at all.

Let us not confuse our need to take restive moments
with laziness or sloth. Rest does not necessarily mean that
we must be confined to bed or become comatose. It can
mean sleeping or walking in the woods. Rest can also
mean working at something we enjoy, like painting a
fence, gardening, or woodworking. The main thing is to

*I enter into nothingness and there
discover everything. Yet I cling to
the illusion of time and space, lest
I disappear. You are in the nothing.*